Keto Life

A Complete Step-by-Step Cooking Guide for Your Daily Low-Carb Diet

Kimberly Wood

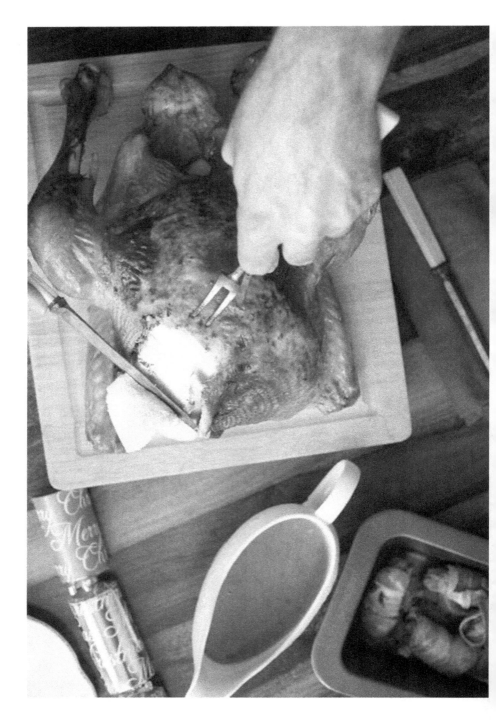

Table of Contents

MEAT

Chicken And Herb Butter With Keto Zucchini Roll-Ups

Macros: Fat 83% | Protein 13% | Carbs 4%

Prep time: 15 minutes | Cook time: 40 minutes | Serves 4

Chicken and herb butter with keto zucchini is the best recipe for a family gathering at dinner, where you find vitamins, protein, and calcium in one dish your child will enjoy a healthy and delicious meal as the family warms up.

ZUCCHINI ROLL-UPS:

- 1½ pounds (680 g) zucchini
- ½ teaspoon salt
- 3 ounces (85 g) butter
- 6 ounces (170 g) mushrooms, finely chopped 6 ounces (170 g) cream cheese
- 6 ounces (170 g) shredded Cheddar cheese
- ½ green bell pepper, chopped
- 2 ounces (57 g) air-dried chorizo, chopped 1 egg
- 1teaspoon onion powder
- 2tablespoons fresh parsley, chopped
- ½ teaspoon salt
- ¼ teaspoon pepper

CHICKEN:

- 4 (6-ounce / 170-g) chicken breasts
- Salt and freshly ground pepper, to taste
- 1 ounce (28 g) butter, for frying

HERB BUTTER:

- 4 ounces (113 g) butter, at room temperature
- 1 garlic clove
- ½ teaspoon garlic powder
- tablespoon fresh parsley, finely chopped
- 1 teaspoon lemon juice
- ½ teaspoon salt

Preheat the oven to 350°F (180°C). Cut the zucchini lengthwise into equal slices, half an inch, Pat dry with paper towels or a clean kitchen towel.and place it on a baking tray lined with parchment paper. Sprinkle salt on the zucchini and let stand for 10 minutes.

Bake for 20 minutes in the oven, or until the zucchini is tender. Transfer to a cooling rack from the oven, Dry more if needed.

Put the butter in the saucepan over medium heat, cut the mushrooms and put it in and stir fry well, let cool.

Add the remaining ingredients for the zucchini roll-ups to a bowl, except a third of the shredded cheese. Add the mushrooms and blend well.

Place a large amount of cheese on top of each zucchini slice.

Roll up and put it inside the baking dish with seams down, Sprinkle on top the remainder of the cheese.

Raise the temperature to 400°F (205°C). Bake for 20 minutes, or until the cheese turns bubbly and golden.

In the meantime, season your chicken and fry it over medium heat in butter until it is crispy on the outside and cooked through.

HERB BUTTER:

To prepare Herb butter mix the butter, garlic, garlic powder, fresh parsley, lemon juice, and salt. thoroughly in a small bowl.

Let sit for 30 minutes and serve on top of the chicken and zucchini roll- ups.

STORAGE: Store in an airtight container in the fridge for up to 5 days or in the freezer for up to 2 weeks.

REHEAT: Microwave, covered, until the desired temperature is reached or reheat in a frying pan.

SERVE IT WITH: Serve with a herb butter or keto-friendly mayonnaise and a green salad.

PER SERVING

calories: 913 | fat: 84.0g | total carbs: 10.0g | fiber: 3.0g | protein: 30.0g

Keto Buffalo Drumsticks With Chili Aioli And Garlic

Macros: Fat 68% | Protein 30% | Carbs 2%

Prep time:10 minutes | Cook time:40 minutes | Serves 4

For those who love chicken with spices, peppers, and olive oil in an easy and simple way, and for those who work all day and want to enjoy a delicious meal, keto buffalo drumsticks with chili aioli and garlic is the best choice for fun and health. It's take 40 minutes to get ready. Cook it and enjoy the taste.

- 2 pounds (907 g) chicken drumsticks or chicken wings

CHILI AIOLI:
- ⅓ cup mayonnaise, keto-friendly
- 1tablespoon smoked paprika powder or smoked chili powder 1 garlic clove, minced
- 2tablespoons olive oil, and more for greasing the baking dish 2 tablespoons white wine vinegar
- 1 teaspoon salt
- 1 teaspoon paprika powder 1 tablespoon tabasco

Preheat the oven to 450°F (235°C).

Make the chili aioli: Combine the mayonnaise, smoked paprika powder, garlic clove, olive oil white wine vinegar, salt, paprika powder and tabasco for the marinade in a small bowl,

Gravy Bacon And Turkey

Macros: Fat 45% | Protein 53% | Carbs 2%

Prep time: 15 minutes | Cook time: 3 hours | Serves 14

This gravy bacon and turkey is very simple to make given that it is made in the same way conventional turkey gravy is made. One extra step is added when making the turkey, which sets this amazing gravy recipe apart!

To my family, it's one of our favorite dishes. I will show you in detail how to make turkey with bacon gravy here.

- 12 pounds (5.4 kg) turkey
- Sea salt and fresh ground black pepper, to taste
- 1 pound (454 g) cherry tomatoes
- 1 cup red onions, diced
- 2 garlic cloves, minced
- 1 large celery stalk, diced
- 4 teaspoons fresh thyme, four small sprigs
- 8 ounces (227 g) bacon (10 slices, diced)
- 8 tablespoons butter
- 2 lemons, the juice
- ⅛ teaspoon guar gum (optional)

SPECIAL EQUIPMENT:

Kitchen twine

Start by preheating the oven to 350°F (180°C).

Remove the neck and giblets from the turkey, pat the turkey dry with paper towels and season both inside and outside of the turkey with salt and pepper.

Insert cherry tomatoes, onions, celery, garlic and thyme into the turkey cavity. Tie the legs together with kitchen twine, and put the turkey on a large roasting pan, tuck its wings under the body.

Cook the bacon in a large skillet over medium heat until crisp, for 7 to 8 minutes. Transfer to paper towels to drain, reserving the drippings in the skillet.

Add the ghee or butter to the skillet with the drippings and stir until melted, then pour into a bowl and stir in the lemon juice. Rub mixture all over the turkey.

Place into oven for 30 minutes. After every 30 minutes, baste the turkey with the drippings. Roast for about 3 hours or until a thermometer inserted into the thigh registers 165°F (74°C).

Remove from oven onto a serving tray to rest for at least 25 minutes before serving.

Meanwhile, pour the drippings into a saucepan. Whisk in the guar gum to thicken, after 2 minutes of whisking, add a touch more if you want a thicker gravy. Then add the reserved bacon for one amazing gravy.

STORAGE: Store in an airtight container in the fridge for up to 5 days. You can freeze the chicken for 1 to 2 months.

REHEAT: Microwave, covered or reheated in a frying pan until the desired temperature is reached.

SERVE IT WITH: Serve the dish with Antipasto Salad and a glass of juice!

PER SERVING

calories: 693 | fat: 35.0g | total carbs: 3.7g | fiber: 0.7g | protein: 86.7g

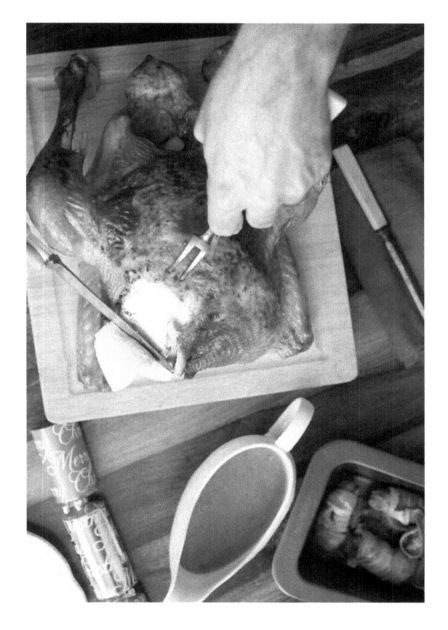

Keto Chicken With Herb Butter

Macros: Fat 82% | Protein 17% | Carbs 1%

Prep time: 10 minutes | Cook time: 10 minutes | Serves 8

There is truly nothing better than a quick, delicious keto chicken with herb butter recipe that gets the dinner on the table in no time. Recipes for fast chicken breasts help me get the dinner on the table fast during the hectic weekends.

This 10-minute keto chicken with herb butter is a true gem and will become a family favorite.

HERB BUTTER:

- 6 ounces (170 g) herb butter, at room temperature
- 1 garlic clove, minced
- ½ teaspoon garlic powder
- ¼ cup fresh parsley, finely chopped
- 1 teaspoon lemon juice
- ½ teaspoon salt

FRIED CHICKEN:

- 3 tablespoons butter
- 4 chicken breasts
- Salt and freshly ground black pepper, to taste

SERVING:

- 8 ounces (227 g) leafy greens (such as baby spinach)

Start with the herb butter. Mix the garlic, parsley, lemon juice and a pinch of salt thoroughly in a small bowl and let sit until it's time to serve.

Cut in half horizontally to make two thin chicken breasts so they cook evenly and quickly. Season the chicken with Italian seasoning, salt, pepper, and crushed red pepper.

Melt the butter over medium heat, in a large frying pan. Put in the chicken and fry in butter until the fillets are cooked through, or a meat thermometer inserted and registers 165°F (75°C). To prevent dry chicken fillets, lower the temperature toward the end.

Serve the chicken on a leafy greens bed and put a generous amount of herb butter over it.

STORAGE: Keep it in the fridge for up to 4 days or in the freezer for up to 1 month.

REHEAT: Reheat it until piping hot throughout. If you're using a microwave, be aware they do not heat evenly throughout, so take your food out halfway through cooking time and give it a stir.

SERVE IT WITH: To make this a complete meal, you can serve it with a side of pasta, veggies, or cauliflower rice.

PER SERVING

calories: 772 | fat: 70.3g | total carbs: 1.5g | fiber: 0.7g | protein: 34.1g

Chicken With Mushrooms And Parmesan Cheese

Macros: Fat 63% | Protein 33% | Carbs 4%

Prep time: 10 minutes | Cook time: 30 minutes | Serves 4

Chicken is always a favorite at week-night. This simple chicken with mushroom and Parmesan cheese features a creamy, cheesy mushroom sauce. It is a quick keto meal, ideal for busy evenings because it can be cooked and prepared in less than 30 minutes.

If you think you don't like mushrooms, think again, because this recipe is about to change the way you feel about mushrooms forever! And if you're already a fan of mushrooms like me and are looking for a way to uplift your game of mushroom-lovin dinner, this recipe has your name all over it.

- 2 tablespoons avocado oil
- 1½ pounds (680 g) boneless chicken thighs
- Salt and freshly ground black pepper, to taste
- 4 garlic cloves, minced
- 8 ounces (227 g) cremini mushrooms, sliced
- 1½ cups heavy whipping cream
- 2 ounces (57 g) Parmesan cheese, grated
- 1 teaspoon fresh parsley

Heat the avocado oil in a large skillet over medium heat. Season the chicken thighs with salt and pepper. Fry in the skillet until browned or cooked; remove the chicken to a slotted spoon plate, conserve the juices

in the pan.

Add garlic to the frying pan and stir-fry until soft; add mushrooms and sauté for around 5 to 7 minutes, until softened.

Put heavy cream on low heat, and stir well. Stirring frequently for about 10 minutes, allow to simmer, incorporate Parmesan cheese to melt. Add salt and chili pepper to taste.

Return the chicken to the skillet and garnish with sauce. Serve with parsley.

STORAGE: Keep a stash of lidded containers so that you have something to store your leftovers in. Use freezer bags if you don't have space to store a lot of containers. Keep it in the fridge for up to 2 to 3 days or in the freezer for up to 3 weeks.

REHEAT: Microwave, covered, or reheated in a frying pan or instant pot, covered, on medium until the desired temperature is reached.

SERVE IT WITH: Serve with a fresh side salad or steamed low-carb vegetables like broccoli, spinach, or asparagus.

PER SERVING

calories: 584 | fat: 41.0g | total carbs: 6.0g | fiber: 0.6g | protein: 48.4g

Chicken With Coconut Curry

Macros: Fat 71% | Protein 22% | Carbs 7%

Prep time: 20 minutes | Cook time: 30 minutes | Serves 6

This flavorful chicken with keto coconut curry recipe is EASY, with a secret trick! You are only 9 ingredients away from low-carbon coconut curry, and 30 minutes away. The easy chicken curry will be a family-wide dinner winner. Plus, it is gluten-free and keto-friendly.

- 2 stalks of lemongrass
- 1½ pounds (680 g) boneless chicken thighs
- 2 tablespoons coconut oil
- 1 tablespoon curry powder
- 1 thumb-sized piece of fresh ginger
- Salt and freshly ground black pepper, to taste
- 1 leek
- 2 garlic cloves
- 1 small red bell pepper, sliced
- ½ red chili pepper, finely chopped
- 14 ounces (397 g) coconut cream
- 1 lemon, zest

Crush the rough part of the lemongrass with the broad side of a knife or a pestle.

Cut the chicken into coarse pieces.

Gently heat the coconut oil in a wok or a large frying pan.

Grate the ginger and fry together with the lemongrass and curry.

Add half of the chicken and sauté over medium heat until the strips are golden. Salt and pepper to taste.

Set aside and fry the rest of the chicken in the same way, perhaps add a little more curry for the second batch. The lemon grass can remain in the pan.

Slice the leek into pieces and sauté them in the same pan together with the other vegetables and the finely chopped garlic. The vegetables should turn golden, but retain their crispiness.

Add the coconut cream and chicken and let simmer for 5 to 10 minutes until everything is warm.

Remove the lemon grass and sprinkle over the lime zest.

STORAGE: Keep your leftovers well sealed and separate. Keeping foods separate and well covered helps to combat potential cross-contamination. store it in a glass or plastic container or to save room for 4 days in the fridge and for 1 month in the freezer, put it into a freezer bag and lay it flat so that it freezes flat.

REHEAT: Microwave, covered, or reheated in a frying pan or instant pot, covered, on medium until the desired temperature is reached. Don't reheat leftovers more than once. This is because the more times you cool and reheat food, the higher the risk of food poisoning.

SERVE IT WITH: Serve with keto eggplant salad with capsicum and a glass of fresh juice.

PER SERVING

calories: 578 | fat: 46.6g | total carbs: 10.8g | fiber: 2.8g | protein: 32.6g

Oven-Baked Chicken In Garlic

Macros: Fat 56% | Protein 43% | Carbs 0%

Prep time: 10 minutes | Cook time: 55 minutes | Serves 4

Looking for a one-pan meal with your family? Or maybe you're just looking for a meal with easy preparation? This oven-baked keto chicken in garlic just needs a big baking dish. It is beautifully flavorful and fragrant. Who knew that a chicken dish would fit into a diet so well?

- 3 pounds (1.4 kg) chicken
- 2 teaspoons sea salt
- ½ teaspoon ground black pepper
- 2 garlic cloves, minced
- 6 ounces (170 g) butter

Preheat the oven to 400°F (205°C). Season the chicken with salt and pepper, both inside and out.

Place chicken breast up in a baking dish.

Combine the garlic and butter in a small saucepan over medium heat. The butter should not turn brown, just melt.

Let the butter cool for a couple of minutes.

Pour the garlic butter over and inside the chicken. Bake on lower oven rack for 1-1 ½ hours, or until internal temperature reaches 180°F (82°C). Baste with the juices from the bottom of the pan every 20 minutes.

Serve with the juices and a side dish of your choice.

STORAGE: Keeping foods separate and well covered helps to combat potential cross-contamination. store it in a plastic container in the fridge for up to 3 to 4 days or in the freezer for up to 3 weeks

REHEAT: Microwave, covered, or reheated in a frying pan or instant pot, covered, on medium until the desired temperature is reached. Don't reheat leftovers more than once. This is because the more times you cool and reheat food, the higher the risk of food poisoning.

SERVE IT WITH: Serve with salad or steamed low-carb vegetables and a glass of fresh juice.

PER SERVING

calories: 686 | fat: 43.7g | total carbs: 0.8g | fiber: 0.1g | protein: 69.7g

Chubby And Juicy Roasted Chicken

Macros: Fat 64% | Protein 34% | Carbs 2%

Prep time: 15 minutes | Cook time: 45 minutes | Serves 4

Thinking of the perfect dish for your special occasion or a simple dinner with the family, palmy roasted chicken is always a crowd-pleaser. Butter, garlic, and lemon give the chicken a rich flavor, while it's cooked away with healthy, aromatic butter or olive oil. Lemon and garlic are just such a wonderful combination!

- 1 teaspoon olive oil
- 1 lemon, zested and cut in half
- ½ tablespoon ground cinnamon
- ½ tablespoon ground ginger
- 3 sprigs fresh thyme, chopped
- 2 sprigs fresh rosemary, chopped
- 2 cloves garlic, minced
- Sea salt and freshly ground black pepper, to taste
- 1 (3-pound / 1.4-kg) whole chicken
- 4 whole garlic cloves
- ¾ cup water

Preheat the oven to 400°F (205°C).

In a bowl, mix together the olive oil, lemon zest, cinnamon, ginger, rosemary, thyme, and minced garlic. To taste, add a pinch salt and pepper.

Rub ⅔ of the mixture over the meat under the skin of the chicken. Stuff the cavity with half of the lemon along with the 4 garlic cloves. This will render the chicken a delicious flavor.

Rub the remaining mixture over the outside of the chicken and season   with salt and pepper.

Arrange the chicken in a roasting pan and pour ¾ cup of water into the pan, Squeeze the juice from the remaining lemon half and rub evenly over the chicken.

Place the chicken in the preheated oven for 45 minutes until completely cooked through and an instant-read thermometer inserted into the thickest part of the thigh, near the bone registers at least 165°F (74°C).

Remove from the oven and cover the pan with a doubled sheet of aluminum foil. Let rest for 5 to 10 minutes before serving.

STORAGE: Store in an airtight container in the fridge for up to 4 days or in the freezer for up to 1 month.

REHEAT: Microwave, covered, until the desired temperature is reached or reheat in a frying pan or air fryer / instant pot, covered, on medium.

SERVE IT WITH: To make this a complete meal, it's best served with Mashed Cauliflower with Parmesan and Chives or Roasted Asparagus with Browned Butter.

PER SERVING

calories: 745 | fat: 52.7g | total carbs: 5.3g | fiber: 1.8g | protein: 64.1g

Baked Pork Gyros

Macros: Fat 61% | Protein 36% | Carbs 3%

Prep time: 6 minutes | Cook time: 25 minutes | Serves 4

Such a delicious and nutritious dish! It has its origin in Greece and is perfect for a quick fix. The best cut of pork to make this dish is the neck or shoulder.

- 1 pound (454 g) ground pork meat
- ½ small chopped onion
- 1 teaspoon ground marjoram
- 1 teaspoon rosemary
- 4 garlic cloves
- ¼ teaspoon black pepper
- ¾ teaspoons salt
- ¾ cup water
- 1 teaspoon dried oregano

Preheat your oven to 400 □ (205 □).

In a food processor, add the ground pork meat, onions, marjoram, rosemary, garlic, black pepper, salt, water, and oregano and process to combine completely.

Tightly press to compact the meat mixture into a loaf pan. Cover with an aluminum foil and poking holes with a toothpick or a fork in the foil.

Bake the loaf in the oven for 25 minutes.

Transfer to a serving platter and serve while warm.

STORAGE: Store in an airtight container in the refrigerator for up to 4 days.

REHEAT: Microwave, covered, until the desired temperature is reached or reheat in a frying pan or air fryer / instant pot, covered, on medium.

SERVE IT WITH: To make this a complete meal, serve with tamari salmon and avocado salad.

PER SERVING

calories: 347 | fat: 23.6g | total carbs: 2.2g | fiber: 0.4g | protein: 29.5g

Coconut Pork Chops

Macros: Fat: 71% | Protein: 26% | Carbs: 3%

Prep time: 10 minutes | Cook time: 27 minutes | Serves 4

A hit recipe of pork chops for the family and a friend's dinner gathering... These fabulous pork chops are so delicious that everyone would love to enjoy it.

- ¼ cup coconut oil, divided
- 1½ pounds (680 g) ¾-inch thick boneless pork chops
  1 tablespoon fresh ginger, grated
- 2teaspoons garlic, minced
- 1 cup unsweetened coconut milk
- 2 tablespoons fresh lime juice
- 1 teaspoon fresh basil, chopped
- ½ cup unsweetened coconut, shredded

In a large nonstick skillet, melt 2 tablespoons of coconut oil over medium heat and cook the pork chops for about 10 minutes, flipping occasionally, or until browned on both sides.

With a spatula, push the pork chops to the side of the skillet. In the center of the wok, add the remaining coconut oil and sauté the ginger and garlic for about 2 minutes. Add the coconut milk, lime juice and basil and stir to combine with the pork chops. Simmer covered for about 12 to 15 minutes.

Remove from the heat to serving plates. Serve with the garnishing of shredded coconut.

STORAGE: Store in an airtight container in the fridge for up to 4 days or in the freezer for up to 1 month.

REHEAT: Microwave, covered, until the desired temperature is reached or reheat in a frying pan or air fryer / instant pot, covered, on medium.

SERVE IT WITH: Enjoy these pork chops with fresh green salad.

PER SERVING

calories: 491 | fat: 39.0g | total carbs: 6.1g | fiber: 3.0g | protein: 32.0g

Bbq Party Pork Kabobs

Macros: Fat: 58% | Protein: 38% | Carbs: 4%

Prep time: 15 minutes | Cook time: 12 minutes | Serves 4

One of the best recipes of pork kabobs that are so juicy and full of flavor. The versatile herbed marinade adds a terrific taste to pork cubes.

- ¼ cup olive oil
- 1 tablespoon garlic, minced
- 2teaspoons dried oregano, crushed
- 1 teaspoon dried parsley, crushed
- 1 teaspoon dried basil, crushed
- Sea salt and ground black pepper, to taste
- 1 (1-pound / 454-g) pork tenderloin, trimmed and cut into 1½-inch pieces
- Olive oil cooking spray

SPECIAL EQUIPMENT:

4 metal skewers

In a mixing bowl, place the oil, garlic, dried herbs, salt, and black pepper and mix well. Add the pork pieces and coat with the marinade generously. Cover the bowl with plastic wrap and refrigerate for 2 to 4 hours.

Preheat your grill to medium-high heat and spray the grill grate with olive oil spray.

Remove the pork pieces from marinade and thread onto 4 metal skewers. Place the pork skewers onto the heated grill and cook for about 12 minutes, flipping occasionally, or until it reach the desired doneness.

Remove the skewers from the grill and place onto a platter for about 5 minutes before serving.

STORAGE: Store in an airtight container in the fridge for up to 4 days or in the freezer for up to 1 month.

REHEAT: Remove the skewers from the freezer and immediately grill, covered, over medium-high heat for about 15 minutes, flipping frequently.

SERVE IT WITH: Serve these pork kabobs over the bed of torn lettuce.

PER SERVING

calories: 261 | fat: 16.7g | total carbs: 2.2g | fiber: 1.0g | protein: 25.0g

One-Pan Sausage & Broccoli

Macros: Fat: 79% | Protein: 17% | Carbs: 4%

Prep time: 10 minutes | Cook time: 20 minutes | Serves 4

A recipe that pairs up the sausage and broccoli for an indulgent meal. This delicious dish is easy to make and everyone will eat it up with happiness.

- 2 tablespoons olive oil
- 1 pound (454 g) mild Italian sausage, casing removed
- 4 cups small broccoli florets
- 1 tablespoon garlic, minced
- Freshly ground black pepper, as required

In a large nonstick skillet, heat the oil over medium heat. Cook the sausage for about 8 to 10 minutes or until browned completely, stirring frequently. With a slotted spoon, transfer the sausage meat onto a plate and set aside.

In the same skillet, add the broccoli and cook for about 6 minutes, stirring frequently. Stir in the garlic and cook for about 3 minutes, stirring frequently. Add the cooked sausage meat and black pepper and cook for about 1 minute.

Remove from the heat and serve hot.

STORAGE: Store in an airtight container in the fridge for up to 4 days or in the freezer for up to 1 month.

REHEAT: Microwave, covered, until the desired temperature is reached or reheat in a frying pan or air fryer / instant pot, covered, on medium.

SERVE IT WITH: Serve this dish with cooked cauliflower rice.

PER SERVING

calories: 487 | fat: 43.2g | total carbs: 7.0g | fiber: 2.0g | protein: 18.9g

Colorful Sausage & Bell Peppers Combo

Macros: Fat: 80% | Protein: 17% | Carbs: 3%

Prep time: 15 minutes | Cook time: 32 minutes | Serves 6

Such a satisfying and colorful combo! With the combo of sweet Italian sausage, bell peppers and onion, this recipe is bursting with delish flavors.

- 1½ pounds (680 g) sweet Italian sausages
- 2 tablespoons olive oil
- 1 red onion, sliced thinly
- 1 orange bell pepper, seeded and cut into 3-inch long strips
- 1 red bell pepper, seeded and cut into 3-inch long strips
- 1 yellow bell pepper, seeded and cut into 3-inch long strips
- 1 tablespoon garlic, minced
- ½ cup white wine
- Sea salt and ground black pepper, to taste
- Olive oil cooking spray

Preheat a grill to medium-high and spray the grill grate with olive oil spray.

Place the sausage links onto the heated grill and cook for about 12 minutes, flipping occasionally. Transfer the sausages onto a plate and set aside for about 15 minutes. Then cut each sausage into 2-inch pieces.

In a large nonstick skillet, heat the oil over medium-high heat and stir in the onion, bell peppers and garlic. Cook for about 10 minutes, stirring occasionally. Add the cooked sausage slices and wine. Cook for about 10 minutes, stirring occasionally. Sprinkle with salt and black pepper to taste.

Remove from the heat and serve hot.

STORAGE: Store in an airtight container in the fridge for up to 4 days or in the freezer for up to 1 month.

REHEAT: Microwave, covered, until the desired temperature is reached or reheat in a frying pan or air fryer / instant pot, covered, on medium.

SERVE IT WITH: Fresh baby spinach goes great with this sausage meal.

TIP: For a nice presentation, cut the bell peppers into uniform slices.

PER SERVING

calories: 450 | fat: 39.9g | total carbs: 5.1g | fiber: 1.0g | protein: 18.0g

Italian Metballs Parmigiana

Macros: Fat: 71% | Protein: 26% | Carbs: 3%

Prep time: 15 minutes | Cook time: 30 minutes | Serves 6

If you're looking for an elegant dish of ground pork, try this rich meatballs recipe! These tender meatballs are smothered in tomato sauce and then topped with Mozzarella cheese.

MEATBALLS:

- 1¼ pounds (567 g) ground pork
- ½ cup Parmesan cheese, shredded
- ½ cup almond flour
- 1 organic egg, beaten lightly
- tablespoon fresh parsley, chopped
- 1 teaspoon fresh oregano, chopped
- 1 teaspoon garlic, minced
- Sea salt and ground black pepper, to taste
- 2 tablespoons olive oil

TOPPING:

- 1 cup sugar-free tomato sauce
- 1 cup Mozzarella cheese, shredded

Preheat the oven 350 ☐ (180°C).

Make the meatballs: In a mixing bowl, add all ingredients except for oil and with your clean hands, mix until well combined. Make about 1½-inch meatballs from the pork mixture. In a large nonstick skillet, heat the oil over medium-high heat and cook the meatballs for about 15 minutes or until cooked through, flipping occasionally.

Remove the meatballs from the heat to a baking dish. Top with the tomato sauce evenly, followed by the Mozzarella cheese. Bake in the preheated oven for about 15 minutes or until the cheese is bubbly and golden.

Remove from the oven and serve hot.

STORAGE: Place the browned and then cooled meatballs in a resealable plastic bag. Seal the bag and freeze for about 3 to 4 days.

REHEAT: Microwave, covered, until the desired temperature is reached or reheat in a frying pan or air fryer / instant pot, covered, on medium.

SERVE IT WITH: Fresh veggie salad accompanies these meatballs nicely.

PER SERVING

calories: 403 | fat: 32.2g | total carbs: 0.9g | fiber: 0g | protein: 26.0g

Spanish Beef Empanadas

Macros: Fat: 78% | Protein: 18% | Carbs: 4%

Prep time: 20 minutes | Cook time: 28 minutes | Serves 6

Make your dinner table more tempting with this cheesy beef empanadas! These delicious empanadas are prepared with a cheesy dough made and spicy beef filling.

DOUGH:

- 1 cup Mozzarella cheese, shredded
- 5 tablespoons cream cheese, softened
- ¾ cup almond flour
- tablespoon coconut flour
- 1 egg, beaten lightly
- tablespoons unsweetened coconut milk
- 1 teaspoon garlic powder
- ½ teaspoon sea salt

FILLING:

- ¼ cup butter
- 1 pound (454 g) ground beef
- 1 onion, chopped
- 1 tablespoon garlic, minced
- 2 teaspoons dried oregano, crushed
- 2 teaspoons ground cumin
- 1 teaspoon chili powder
- Sea salt and freshly ground black pepper, to taste

Make the dough: In a small nonstick saucepan, add the Mozzarella and cream cheese over low heat and cook for about 2 to 3 minutes or until melted, stirring occasionally.

Remove from the heat to a heatproof mixing bowl. In the bowl of cheese mixture, add the flours, egg, coconut milk, garlic powder and salt. Mix well until a dough ball forms. Cover the bowl with plastic wrap, and then press it down slightly onto the surface of the dough. Refrigerate the bowl for about 30 minutes.

Make the filling: In a large nonstick skillet, melt the butter over medium- high heat and cook the beef for about 7 minutes until browned, breaking up the lumps of meat with a spatula. Add the onion and garlic and cook for about 4 to 5 minutes. Stir in the oregano, cumin, chili powder, salt and black pepper. Mix well and remove from the heat. Set the beef mixture aside to cool completely.

Preheat the oven to 425 □ (220°C) and line a baking sheet with parchment paper.

Make the empanadas: Arrange a parchment paper on a flat surface. Place the dough over the parchment paper and with your hands, press into a thin layer. With a 3-inch round cutter, cut the dough into 12 circles. With a spoon, place the filling into the center of 1 dough circle. Fold the dough over and with a fork, then press the edges together to seal the filling. Repeat with remaining empanadas.

Arrange the empanadas on the prepared baking sheet in a single layer.

Bake for about 10 to 12 minutes or until golden brown.

Remove the empanadas from the oven and serve on plates.

STORAGE: The assembled but unbaked empanadas can be covered in plastic and stored in the fridge for up to 2 days.

REHEAT: Microwave, covered, until the desired temperature is reached or reheat in a frying pan or air fryer / instant pot, covered, on medium.

SERVE IT WITH: Serve these empanadas with low-carb dressing.

PER SERVING

calories: 436 | fat: 38.1g | total carbs: 3.9g | fiber: 1.0g | protein: 19.0g

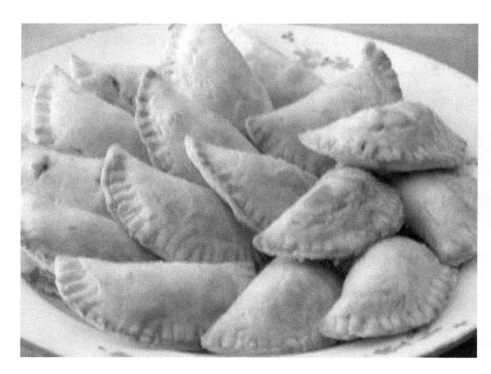

FISH

Low Carb Seafood Chowder

Macros: Fat 66% | Protein 26% | Carbs 8%

Prep time: 20 minutes | Cook time: 20 minutes | Serves 4

You have no time to prepare a great meal for your friends and guests. Here's the low-carb seafood chowder, a perfect rich recipe that you can prepare it in minimal time. Let your guests relish during the day.

- 4 tablespoons butter
- 5 ounces (142 g) celery stalks, sliced
- 2 garlic cloves, minced
- 4 ounces (113 g) cream cheese
- 1 cup clam juice
- 1½ cups heavy whipping cream
- 2 teaspoons dried sage or dried thyme
- ½ lemon, juiced and zested
- 1 pound (454 g) salmon fillets, cut into 1-inch pieces
- 8 ounces (227 g) shrimp, peeled and deveined
- 2 ounces (57 g) baby spinach
- Salt and freshly ground black pepper, to taste Fresh sage, for garnish

Melt the butter in a large pot over medium heat. Add celery and garlic. Cook for about 5 minutes, stirring occasionally. Add clam juice, cream, cream cheese, sage, lemon juice and lemon zest. Let it simmer for about 10 minutes without a lid.

Add the salmon and shrimp. Simmer for 3 minutes or until salmon is opaque. Add the baby spinach and stir until wilted. Season with salt and pepper.

Garnish with fresh sage before serving for extra flavor.

STORAGE: The rest of the mixture can be kept in an airtight container in the fridge for 4 days, and it can also be kept in the freezer for 10 days.

REHEAT: Microwave, covered, until the desired temperature is reached or reheat in a frying pan or instant pot, covered, on medium.

SERVE IT WITH: You can serve this recipe with keto sesame salmon and cucumber and fennel salad.

PER SERVING

calories: 622 | fat: 46.7g | total carbs: 12.5g | fiber: 1.6g | protein: 38.8g

Keto Chili-Covered Salmon with Spinach

Macros: Fat 55% | Protein 38% | Carbs 7%

Prep time: 5 minutes | Cook time: 20 minutes | Serves 4

This chili-covered salmon with spinach is elegant, spicy, easy, delicious, and keto. What more can you want out of dinner?

- ¼ cup olive oil
- 1½ pounds (680 g) salmon, in pieces
- Salt and freshly ground black pepper, to taste
- 1 ounce (28 g) Parmesan cheese, grated finely
- 1 tablespoon chili paste
- ½ cup sour cream
- 1 pound (454 g) fresh spinach

Preheat oven to 400°F (205°C).

Grease the baking dish with half of the olive oil, season the salmon with pepper and salt, and put in the baking dish, skin-side down.

Combine Parmesan cheese, chili paste and sour cream. Then spread them on the salmon fillets.

Bake for 20 minutes, or until the salmon flakes easily with a fork or it becomes opaque.

Heat the remaining olive oil in a nonstick skillet, sauté the spinach until it's wilted, about a couple of minutes, and season with pepper and salt.

Serve with the oven-baked salmon immediately.

STORAGE: This recipe is freezer friendly, so it can be stored in the freezer for up to 3 months. To freeze, cover each quiche slice tightly in aluminum foil and freeze for up to 3 months.

REHEAT: Place it in the microwave until the desired temperature, or reheat in a frying pan.

SERVE IT WITH: To make this a complete meal, serve with riced cauliflower and a green salad.

PER SERVING

calories: 461 | fat: 28.5g | total carbs: 8.0g | fiber: 2.8g | protein: 42.6g

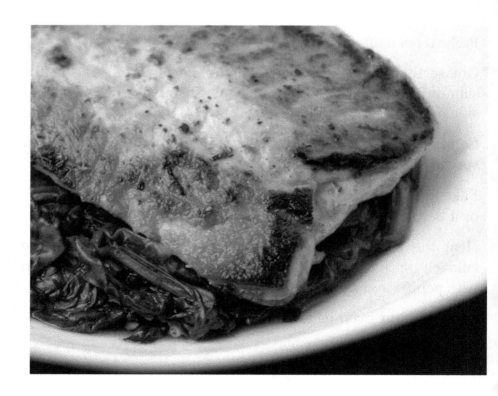

Keto Egg Butter with Avocado and Smoked Salmon

Macros: Fat 84% | Protein 11% | Carbs 5%

Prep time: 5 minutes | Cook time: 15 minutes | Serves 4

This is what we call a breakfast for champions! If you want a keto meal that will keep you on top of your game for hours and hours, this is it!

- 4 eggs
- ½ teaspoon sea salt
- ¼ teaspoon ground black pepper
- 5 ounces (142 g) butter, at room temperature
- 4 ounces (113 g) smoked salmon
- 1 tablespoon fresh parsley, chopped finely
- 2 avocados
- 2 tablespoons olive oil

Put the eggs in a pot and cover them with cold water. Then put the pot on the stove without a lid and bring it to a boil.

Lower the heat and let it simmer for 6 to 9 minutes. Then remove eggs from the water and put them in a bowl with cold water.

Peel the eggs and cut them finely. Use a fork to mix the eggs and butter.

Then season to taste with pepper, salt.

Serve the egg butter with slices of smoked salmon, finely chopped parsley, and a side of diced avocado tossed in olive oil.

STORAGE: Store in an airtight container in the fridge for up to 2 days.

REHEAT: Place it in the microwave until it reaches the desired temperature.

SERVE IT WITH: To make this a complete meal, serve with cauliflower rice and a green salad.

PER SERVING

calories: 638 | fat: 61.1g | total carbs: 9.8g | fiber: 6.8g | protein: 16.5g

Keto Baked Salmon with Butter And Lemon Slices

Macros: Fat 71% | Protein 29% | Carbs 0%

Prep time: 10 minutes | Cook time: 25 minutes | Serves 6

This lemon salmon is out-of-this-world delicious. With only a few ingredients, it's easy and quick to make. This lemon butter sauce and salmon recipe is good enough for company but easy enough for a weeknight dinner!

- 1 tablespoon olive oil
- 2 pounds (907 g) salmon
- 1 teaspoon sea salt
- Freshly ground black pepper, to taste
- 7 ounces (198 g) butter
- 1 lemon

Start by preheating the oven to 425°F (220°C).

In a large baking dish, spray it with olive oil. Then add the salmon, skin- side down. Season with salt and pepper.

Cut the lemon into thin slices and place them on the upper side of the salmon. Cut the butter in thin slices and spread them on top of the lemon slices.

Put the dish in the heated oven and bake on the middle rack for about 25 to 30 minutes, or until the salmon flakes easily with a fork.

Melt the rest of the butter in a small saucepan until it bubbles. Then remove from heat and let cool a little. Consider adding some lemon juice on the melted cool butter.

Serve the fish with the lemon butter.

STORAGE: Store in an airtight container in the fridge for up to 2 days.

REHEAT: Microwave, covered, until the desired temperature is reached or reheat in a frying pan or air fryer / instant pot, covered, on medium.

SERVE IT WITH: To make this a complete meal, serve with riced broccoli and a green salad.

PER SERVING

calories: 474 | fat: 37.6g | total carbs: 0.7g | fiber: 0.1g | protein: 32.6g

Grilled Tuna Salad with Garlic Sauce

Macros: Fat 61% | Protein 31% | Carbs 8%

Prep time: 10 minutes | Cook time: 15 minutes | Serves 4

A crisp, pretty salad topped with grilled tuna. Our creamy garlic dressing pulls it all together. It's simple to make so you can enjoy a tasty keto meal and the warm sunshine!

GARLIC DRESSING:

- ⅔ cup keto-friendly mayonnaise
- 2 tablespoons water
- 2 teaspoons garlic powder
- Salt and freshly ground black pepper, to taste

TUNA SALAD:

- 2 eggs
- 8 ounces (227 g) green asparagus
- 1 tablespoon olive oil
- ¾ pound (340 g) fresh tuna, in slices
- 4 ounces (113 g) leafy greens
- 2 ounces (57 g) cherry tomatoes
- ½ red onion
- 2 tablespoons pumpkin seeds
- Salt and freshly ground black pepper, to taste

Mix the ingredients together for the garlic dressing. And set them aside.

Put the eggs in boiling water for 8 to 10 minutes. Cooling in cold water would facilitate the peeling.

Slice the asparagus into lengths and rapidly fry them inside a hot pan with no oil or butter. Then set them aside.

Rub the tuna with oil and fry or grill for 2 to 3 minutes on each side.

Season with salt and pepper.

Put the leafy greens, asparagus, peeled eggs cut in halves, tomatoes and thinly sliced onion into a plate.

Finally, cut the tuna into slices and spread the slices evenly over the salad. Pour the dressing on top and add some pumpkin seeds.

STORAGE: Store in an airtight container in the fridge for up 2 to 4 days.

SERVE IT WITH: To make this a complete meal, serve with a roasted chicken thigh.

PER SERVING

calories: 397 | fat: 27.1g | total carbs: 8.3g | fiber: 2.8g | protein: 30.0g

Crispy Keto Creamy Fish Casserole

Macros: Fat 70% | Protein 23% | Carbs 8%

Prep time: 25 minutes | Cook time: 30 minutes | Serves 4

Once you finish your hard work, you need a crunchy meal to indulge yourself with. Crispy keto creamy fish casserole will hit the spot as it's so easy to make by yourself. With a few ingredients, you will get this fabulous dish!

- 1 head broccoli, cut into florets
- 2 tablespoons olive oil
- 1 teaspoon salt
- ¼ teaspoon freshly ground black pepper
- 6 scallions, chopped
- 1 ounce (28 g) melted butter, for greasing the casserole dish
- 1 tablespoon parsley, finely chopped
- 1¼ cups heavy whipping cream
- 1 tablespoon Dijon mustard
- 1½ pounds (680 g) white fish, in serving- pieces
- 3 ounces (85 g) butter slices, under room temperature

Preheat the oven to 400 □ (205°C).

Heat the olive oil in a nonstick skillet over medium heat.

Add the broccoli to the skillet and sauté for 5 to 7 minutes or until tender, then season the broccoli with salt and ground black pepper, add the finely chopped scallions, and sauté for 1 to 2 minutes more.

Prepare a casserole dish and grease it with butter to add a tasty level of flavors to the meal. Then pour the sautéed broccoli and scallions in the casserole dish, stir them well until they have a delicious butter smell.

In a bowl, mix finely chopped parsley with cream and Dijon mustard and pour the mixture over the casserole dish. Stir until fully incorporated.

Then nestle the white fish in the casserole dish. Top them with the butter slices.

Cook in the preheated oven for 20 to 30 minutes, or until the fish exudes tender and takes in the flavor from the delicious butter.

Remove the casserole dish from the oven and serve the fish and vegetables warm.

STORAGE: We can store the leftovers in an airtight container in the freezer for up to 4 days. Use it as a side dish in the coming days.

REHEAT: Reheat the recipe by wrapping the leftovers in aluminum foil and reheating in the oven for 5 to 7 minutes.

SERVE IT WITH: Serve it warm with creamy spinach and dill or with fresh salad to enjoy your meal to utmost.

PER SERVING

calories: 611 | fat: 48.3g | total carbs: 13.2g | fiber: 4.8g | protein: 34.4g

Coconut Keto Salmon and Napa Cabbage

Macros: Fat 74% | Protein 22% | Carbs 4%

Prep time: 10 minutes | Cook time: 20 minutes | Serves 4

The soft palate of shredded coconut combines with tender salmon. This dish will bring you a delightful experience of eating. Simple but crisp taste of Napa cabbage, and this recipe embraces all the nutrients you need.

- 1¼ pounds (567 g) salmon
- 1 tablespoon coconut oil
- 1 teaspoon sea salt
- ½ teaspoon onion powder
- 1 teaspoon turmeric
- 2 ounces (57 g) unsweetened shredded coconut
- 4 tablespoons olive oil, for frying
- 1¼ pounds (567 g) Napa cabbage
- Salt and freshly ground black pepper, to taste
- 4 ounces (113 g) butter
- Lemon, for serving

On a wooden board, cut the salmon into 1×1-inch pieces. Then rub coconut oil on salmon pieces. Place the pieces in a medium bowl and set aside.

Prepare a mixture of salt, onion powder, turmeric, and unsweetened shredded coconut, finely mix the mixture. Meanwhile, put the salmon pieces into this creamy mixture to get a good coating.

In a nonstick frying pan with 4 tablespoons of olive oil on medium heat.

Fry the seasoned salmon pieces with coconut mixture for about 4 to 7 minutes in a pan, stirring every 2 minutes. Leave it in the pan until golden brown, or until soft.

Meanwhile, prepare and cut the cabbage into wedges. Fry the cabbage in a saucepan with butter until it turns into a light creamy liquid. On a platter, pour the cabbage liquid and generously season with salt and pepper.

In a dish decorated with lemon slices, place the fried salmon and pour the creamy cabbage liquid and top with wedges of lemon. Serve warm!

STORAGE: Store in an airtight container in the fridge for up to 4 days or in the freezer for up to 1 month.

REHEAT: You can reheat the extras smoothly in a light skillet on medium- low heat until warmed through.

SERVE IT WITH: Serve it immediately with vegetable soup or crispy salad to be a perfect meal. Enjoy to the full!

PER SERVING

calories: 628 | fat: 52.9g | total carbs: 7.1g | fiber: 1.6g | protein: 32.7g

SOUPS

Spicy Pork and Spinach Stew

Macros: Fat 44% | Protein 46% | Carbs 10%

Prep time: 5 minutes | Cook time: 40 minutes | Serves 4

Everyone will surprise once you make this quick and hearty weeknight dinner fare, loaded to the brim with tender pork stew, spinach and Cajun seasoning along with the onion. I think everyone will ask for seconds. Since it is made in a pressure cooker, you can make it with minimal effort but still have so much flavour.

- 4 garlic cloves
- 1 large onion
- 1pound (454 g) pork butt meat cut into 2-inch chunks
- 1 teaspoon dried thyme
- 2 teaspoons Cajun seasoning blend
- ½ cup heavy whipping cream
- 4 cups baby spinach, chopped

Place garlic and onion in the blender and process until smooth. Pour the purée to the pressure cooker.

Then, add the pork, thyme, and the Cajun seasoning to it. Mix and seal the lid.

Press the 'manual' or 'pressure button' and set the timer to 20 minutes.

Once the time is up, allow the pressure to release naturally for 10 minutes.

Carefully open the lid and stir in the cream and spinach.

Select the 'sauté' button and cook for 5 minutes until the spinach is wilted.

Transfer to a serving bowl and enjoy it hot.

STORAGE: Store in an airtight container in the refrigerator for up to 3 days or the freezer for up to 3 months.

REHEAT: Microwave, covered, until the desired temperature is reached or reheat in a pan / instant pot, covered, on low.

SERVE IT WITH: To make this a complete meal, serve the soup along with a broccoli salad, or riced cauliflower.

PER SERVING

calories: 230 | fat: 11.2g | total carbs: 6.9g | fiber: 1.2g | protein: 31.4g

Lamb Soup

Macros: Fat 72% | Protein 19% | Carbs 9%

Prep time: 5 minutes | Cook time: 25 minutes | Serves 6

This soup has an abundance of flavor. Between the red chili paste, coconut milk, lime juice, and garlic, your taste buds are sure to tingle. What's more, the soup is super-quick, easy to make. And all these makes it a fantastic, comforting lunch or dinner.

- 1 tablespoon coconut oil
- 12 ounces (340 g) ground lamb
- ½ chopped onion
- 2 teaspoons minced garlic
- 2 cups shredded cabbage
- 4 cups chicken broth
- 1½ tablespoons red chili paste
- 2 cups unsweetened coconut milk
- Zest and juice of 1 lime
- 1 cup shredded kale

Heat coconut oil in a medium stockpot over medium-high heat and then stir in the lamb.

Cook for 5 minutes or until browned while stirring the lamb continuously.

Stir in onion, garlic, and cabbage to it and sauté for 4 minutes or until softened.

Pour the chicken broth, red chili paste, coconut milk, lime juice, and lime zest. Mix to combine well.

Then, bring them to a boil and turn the heat to low. Simmer for further 8 minutes until the cabbage is tender.

Add the kale and stir for 3 minutes until wilted.

Transfer to a serving bowl and serve it hot.

STORAGE: Store in an airtight container in the refrigerator for up to 3 days or the freezer for up to 3 months.

REHEAT: Microwave, covered, until the desired temperature is reached or reheat in a pan / instant pot, covered, on low.

SERVE IT WITH: To make this a complete meal, serve the soup along with cauliflower rice or roasted Brussels sprouts.

PER SERVING

calories: 326 | fat: 26.1g | total carbs: 9.3g | fiber: 1.7g | protein: 15.2g

New England Clam Chowder

Macros: Fat 57% | Protein 30% | Carbs 13%

Prep time: 10 minutes | Cook time: 30 minutes | Serves 8

This classic comfort food comes your way through this easy-to-make recipe which can be made in less than 40 minutes. Jam-packed with delectable clams, salty bacon, and hearty celery, this creamy, rich clam chowder will become your new family favorite fare. If you want to make the chowder thicker and indulgent, you can substitute the heavy cream with mascarpone cheese.

- 4 ounces (113 g) uncured bacon, chopped
- 2 tablespoons grass-fed butter
- ½ finely chopped onion
- 2 teaspoons minced garlic
- 1 celery stalk, chopped
- 2 tablespoons arrowroot powder
- 4 cups fish or chicken stock
- 2 bay leaves
- 1 teaspoon chopped fresh thyme
- 1½ cups heavy whipping cream
- 3 (6½-ounce / 185-g) cans clams, drained
- Sea salt, for seasoning
- Freshly ground black pepper, for seasoning
- 2 tablespoons chopped fresh parsley

Fry bacon in a medium stockpot over medium heat till crispy. With a slotted spoon, transfer the bacon to a plate. Keep it aside.

Spoon in butter to sauté the onion, garlic, and celery for 3 minutes.

Add the arrowroot powder and sauté for a minute.

Pour the fish stock, bay leaves, and thyme over it. Bring the mixture to just before it boils.

Lower the heat to medium-low and simmer for 9 minutes or until thickened.

Add the heavy cream and clams. Stir and simmer for further 4 minutes or till heated through.

Discard the bay leaves and sprinkle with salt and pepper.

Transfer to a serving bowl and top it with parsley and crumbled bacon.

Serve hot.

STORAGE: Store in an airtight container in the refrigerator for up to 3days. If you need to freeze, then stop the cooking process at step 5. When you need to serve the chowder, take it out and stir the clams and heavy cream to it.

REHEAT: Microwave, covered with a plastic wrap, for 3 to 4 minutes at high power while stirring it once halfway or reheat in a pan, covered, on medium.

SERVE IT WITH: To make this a complete meal, serve the soup along with oyster crackers or with cauliflower rice.

PER SERVING

calories: 225 | fat: 14.3g | fiber: 8.1g | fiber: 0.7g | protein: 16.7g

Creamy Spinach Soup

Macros: Fat 83% | Protein 4% | Carbs 13%

Prep time: 5 minutes | Cook time: 15 minutes | Serves 2

Wonderfully nutritious and delicious, this vibrant green soup is the perfect evening snack or as the starter for your dinner. Furthermore, the soup is a never-fail recipe. If you love crispy bacon and Parmesan cheese, go wild and add those as toppings to make it more flavorful.

- 1 tablespoon butter
- 1 (2-ounce / 57-g) small onion, sliced
- 2 (½-ounce / 14-g) medium garlic cloves, finely minced 1½ cups water
- ⅔ cup chopped spinach
- 1 chicken stock cube
- ½ cup heavy whipping cream

Heat a saucepan and melt the butter over medium heat.

Add onion to it and cook till softened. Stir in the garlic and keep cooking.

Once the onion is browned, pour half the water along with spinach and stock cube.

Cover and continue cooking until the spinach has wilted.

Transfer the mixture in the saucepan to a blender and pulse until smooth and silky.

Pass it through a fine sieve and add the remaining water according to your desired consistency.

Return to the saucepan and heat it through. Off the heat and stir in the cream.

Pour the soup to the bowl and serve warm.

STORAGE: Store in an airtight container in the refrigerator for up to 3 days or the freezer for up to 3 months.

REHEAT: Microwave, covered, until the desired temperature is reached or reheat in a pan / instant pot, covered, on low.

SERVE IT WITH: To make this a complete meal, you can top it with pepper slices and toasted nuts, then pair it with grilled chicken or fish.

PER SERVING

calories: 185 | fat: 19.1g | total carb: 6.0g | fiber: 6.7g | protein: 1.9g

Sour Garlic Zucchini Soup

Macros: Fat: 79% | Protein: 5% | Carbs: 16%

Prep time: 13 minutes | Cook time: 27 minutes | Serves 2

This sour garlic zucchini soup dish perfectly combines delicious bone broth and that tasty zucchini. It is quick and easy to make and is perfect for cold nights or if you just have the flu. Grab a spoon and get cooking!

- 2 small zucchinis, chopped
- 2 tablespoons olive oil
- 1 small onion peeled and grated
- 2 garlic cloves, minced
- ½ teaspoon of sea salt
- ¼ teaspoon black pepper
- ¼ teaspoon poultry seasoning
- 1½ cups beef bone broth
- 1 small lemon, juiced
- 5 tablespoons sour cream

Pour some water into a medium-sized pan, then add the zucchini and bring it to a boil over medium heat.

Reduce the heat to low and let it simmer for 20 minutes, then drain the zucchini and set aside.

In a small saucepan, put the olive oil, onions, garlic, salt, black pepper, and poultry seasoning, then let it cook for 2 minutes. Pour the beef bone broth into the pan and simmer on low heat for 5 minutes.

Add the lemon juice, then pour the mixture into a blender and blend until it is smooth.

Top the soup with sour cream and serve hot.

STORAGE: Store in an airtight container in the fridge for up to 4 days or in the freezer for up to 1 month.

REHEAT: Microwave, covered, until the desired temperature is reached or reheat in a frying pan or instant pot, covered, on medium.

SERVE IT WITH: To make this a complete meal, serve it with garlicky roasted broccoli.

PER SERVING

calories: 199 | fat: 17.0g | total carbs: 9.1g | fiber: 1.0g | protein: 2.5g

Green Garlic and Cauliflower Soup

Macros: Fat: 56% | Protein: 14% | Carbs: 30%

Prep time: 7 minutes | Cook time: 13 minutes | Serves 5

This garlic and cauliflower soup is a delicious, healthy substitute for potato soup. It is quick and easy to make, but that does not affect the delicious taste of the soup. Comfort your loved ones with this green garlic and cauliflower soup to remind them of all the love that comes from your kitchen. The carbs in this recipe is relatively high, but you can control the content of the carbs by using homemade low-carb vegetable soup.

- 2 teaspoons thyme powder
- 3 cups vegetable soup
- ½ teaspoon matcha green tea powder
- 1 head cauliflower
- 3 tablespoons olive oil
- 5 garlic cloves chopped
- Salt and freshly ground black pepper, to taste

SPECIAL EQUIPMENT:

Immersion blender

Pour the thyme powder, vegetable soup, and the matcha green tea powder into a large pot over medium-high heat. Let it boil for 1 minute.

Add the cauliflower and let it cook for 10 minutes.

Meanwhile, in a small saucepan, add the olive oil and the garlic, then let it cook for 1 minute. Pour it into the pot with the cauliflower. Season with salt and pepper and cook for another 2 minutes.

Put an immersion blender into the pot and purée it until it is smooth.

Remove from the heat and serve while it still warm.

STORAGE: Store in an airtight container in the fridge for up to 4 days or in the freezer for up to 1 month.

REHEAT: Microwave, covered, until the desired temperature is reached or reheat in a frying pan or instant pot, covered, on medium.

SERVE IT WITH: To make this a complete meal, serve it with a bowl of salad.

PER SERVING

calories: 156 | fat: 9.7g | total carbs: 16.1g | fiber: 4.3g | protein: 5.3g

Sour Chicken and Kale Soup

Macros: Fat: 51% | Protein: 42% | Carbs: 7%

Prep time: 7 minutes | Cook time: 13 minutes | Serves 6

This is the chicken soup that satisfies all cravings. This delicious chicken kale soup has the perfect tanginess that keeps you awake when eating with the delicious juiciness of the chicken and kale. It is a perfect leftover dish and helps with cleansing your body and boosting your immune system.

- 2 pounds (907 g) chicken breast, skinless
- Salt and freshly ground black pepper, to taste
- 1 tablespoon olive oil
- ⅓ cup onion
- 14 ounces (397 g) chicken bone broth
- ½ cup olive oil
- 4 cups chicken stock
- ¼ cup lemon juice
- 5 ounces (142 g) baby kale leaves

Sprinkle the chicken with salt and pepper and set aside.

Pour the olive oil and onion into a pan over medium heat and lay the chicken on the pan. Reduce the temperature and let it fry for 15 minutes on both sides.

Remove the chicken from pan and put on a plate, then use a fork to shred the chicken and put it in a blender.

Pour the chicken bone broth into the blender and pulse until it is smooth.

Pour the puréed chicken into the crockpot and add the remaining olive oil, chicken stock, lemon juice, and baby kale leaves.

Allow to simmer on low, covered, for 6 hours stirring once in a while until the soup has thickened.

Remove from the heat and serve hot.

STORAGE: Store in an airtight container in the fridge for up to 4 days or in the freezer for up to 1 month.

REHEAT: Microwave, covered, until the desired temperature is reached or reheat in a frying pan or instant pot, covered, on medium.

SERVE IT WITH: To make this a complete meal, serve it with some Parmesan roasted zucchini.

PER SERVING

calories: 496 | fat: 28.0g | total carbs: 9.4g | fiber: 1.0g | protein: 52.5g

APPETIZERS

Crab–Stuffed Avocado

Macros: Fat 72% | Protein 17% | Carbs 11%

Prep time: 20 minutes | Cook time: 0 minutes | Serves 2

Crab-stuffed avocado salad is an amazingly delicious dish suitable for a light lunch. The meal is healthy, scrumptious, and filing. The stuffed crab goes well with the nutritive avocado.

- 1 halved lengthwise avocado, peeled and pitted
- ½ teaspoon freshly squeezed lemon juice
- 4½ ounces (127 g) Dungeness crab meat
- ¼ cup English cucumber, peeled and chopped
- ¼ cup red bell pepper, chopped
- ½ cup cream cheese
- 1 teaspoon cilantro, chopped
- ½ scallion, chopped
- Sea salt and freshly ground black pepper, to taste

Brush the avocado edges with lemon juice, then set in a bowl.

In a bowl, add the crab meat, cucumber, red pepper, cream cheese, cilantro, scallion, salt, and pepper then stir to mix.

Divide the crab meat mixture in the avocado halves before serving.

STORAGE: Store in an airtight container in the fridge for up to 4 days or in the freezer for up to 1 month.

SERVE IT WITH: To make this a complete meal, serve the dish on a bed of greens.

PER SERVING

calories: 420 | fat: 32.0g | total carbs: 12.6g | fiber: 7.0g | protein: 16.8g

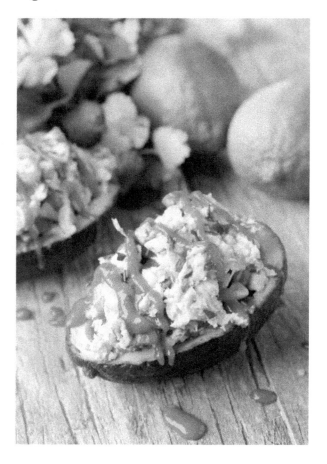

Cheddar Cheese Jalapeño Poppers

Macros: Fat 83% | Protein 13% | Carbs 4%

Prep time: 15 minutes | Cook time: 20 minutes | Serves 3

Jalapeño poppers require few ingredients mainly bacon, jalapeño peppers and shredded Cheddar cheese. The yummy treat takes a short time to prepare.

- 5 slices bacon
- 6 jalapeño peppers
- 3 ounces (85 g) softened cream cheese
- ¼ teaspoon garlic powder
- ¼ cup Cheddar cheese, shredded

In a skillet over medium-high heat, add the bacon and fry for 3 to 4 minutes on each side until crispy. Allow the bacon to cool on a paper towel-lined plate.

Chop the bacon into ½-inch pieces.

Preheat the oven to 400°F (205°C) and line a rimmed baking sheet with parchment paper.

Slice the jalapeño peppers into halves. Using a spoon, scrap out the membranes and seeds.

In a bowl, use a fork to mix the cream cheese, garlic powder, Cheddar cheese, and bacon bits. Spoon the mixture into every jalapeño half, then arrange them on the lined baking sheet.

Bake in the preheated oven until the cheese melts for about 20 minutes and slightly crispy on top.

Transfer to serving plates to cool before serving.

STORAGE: Store in an airtight container in the fridge for up to 4 days or in the freezer for up to 1 month.

REHEAT: Microwave, covered, until it reaches the desired temperature.

SERVE IT WITH: To make this a complete meal, serve with a cup of zoodles or kelp pasta.

PER SERVING

calories: 314 | fat: 16.2g | total carbs: 3.5g | fiber: 0.8g | protein: 10.4g

Crispy Chicken

Macros: Fat 67% | Protein 32% | Carbs 2%

Prep time: 2 minutes | Cook time: 20 minutes | Serves 12

Chicken crisps are naturally crunchy dish that can be served for dinner. The meal is protein packed and takes a very short time to prepare. Everyone in the family will love it.

- 12 (9-ounces / 255-g) chicken thigh skins

SEASONING:

- 3 tablespoons coriander, ground
- 2 tablespoons gray sea salt, finely ground
- 1¼ teaspoons turmeric powder
- ¾ teaspoon celery seed, ground
- ¾ teaspoon parsley, dried
- 2 teaspoons mustard, ground
- 2 tablespoons onion powder
- 2 teaspoons paprika
- ½ teaspoon black pepper, ground

Preheat the oven to 325°F (160°C) and line a rimmed baking sheet with parchment paper.

Cut another parchment paper similar in size to the above and have a separate smaller baking sheet so you can nestle the smaller baking sheet inside the bigger baking sheet.

Make the seasoning: In a ½-cup glass jar, add the coriander, salt, turmeric, celery, parsley, mustard, onion powder, paprika, and black pepper. Cover the jar, then shake.

In a bowl, transfer the chicken skins, then sprinkle 1 tablespoon of the seasoning. Toss until the skins are coated evenly.

On the larger baking sheet, arrange the skins evenly by placing them close.

Set the second parchment paper on the skins, then top with the smaller baking sheet to force the skins to remain in flattened state throughout the baking process.

Bake in the preheated oven until crispy for 20 minutes. Flip the chicken thigh skins halfway through.

Transfer the crisp chicken skins to serving plates to cool before serving.

STORAGE: Store in an airtight container in the fridge for up to 5 days or in the freezer for up to 1 month.

REHEAT: You can remove them from the freezer and enjoy immediately, or microwave, covered, until it reaches the desired temperature.

SERVE IT WITH: To make this a complete meal, serve with broccoli chowder soup.

PER SERVING

calories: 434 | fat: 32.2g | total carbs: 2.0g | fiber: 0.5g | protein: 32.2g

Easy Parmesan Chive and Garlic Crackers

4 Macros: Fat 72% | Protein 16% | Carbs 12%

Prep time: 40 minutes | Cook time: 15 minutes| Serves

Parmesan chive and garlic crackers are perfect for holiday nights and weekday dinners. They are also perfect low-carb snacks for keto diet. The recipe is super easy and produces amazing results.

- 1 tablespoon olive oil
- 1 cup Parmesan cheese, finely grated
- ¼ cup chives, chopped
- 1 cup almond flour, blanched
- ½ teaspoon garlic powder
- 1 large egg, whisked
- 1 tablespoon butter, melted

SPECIAL EQUIPMENT:

A pastry cutter

Preheat the oven to 350°F (180°C) and grease 2 large baking sheets with 1 tablespoon olive oil each.

In a bowl, add the cheese, chives, almond flour, and garlic powder and mix well to combine.

In another bowl, add the eggs and butter, then whisk them well.

Pour the egg mixture into the cheese mixture and blend well until you form a dough.

Divide dough into two equal portions and press well until they are ¼ inch thick.

Use a pastry cutter to slice each dough sheet into 25 equally sized crackers.

Lay the crackers onto the prepared baking sheets.

Bake in the preheated oven for 15 minutes until crispy. Turn off the oven and let the crackers rest for a few minutes before serving.

STORAGE: Store in an airtight container in the fridge for up to 4 days or in the freezer for up to 1 month.

REHEAT: Microwave, covered, until it reaches the desired temperature.

SERVE IT WITH: To make this a complete meal, serve with a cup of plain Greek yogurt.

PER SERVING

calories: 313 | fat: 26.4g | total carbs: 9.0g | fiber: 3.0g | protein: 12.9g

Low Carb Keto Sausage Balls

Macros: Fat 80% | Protein 17% | Carbs 4%

Prep time: 30 minutes | Cook time: 20 minutes | Serves 6

The keto sausage balls are the ideal low-carb snacks for various occasions. These sausage balls offer the best appetizers. The recipe has easy steps that make the snack simple to prepare.

- 2 tablespoons olive oil
- 1 cup almond flour, blanched
- 1 pound (454 g) bulk Italian sausage
- 1¼ cups shredded sharp Cheddar cheese
- 2 teaspoons baking powder
- 1 large beaten egg

Preheat the oven to 350°F (180°C) and grease a baking sheet with olive oil.

In a bowl, mix the flour, sausage, cheese, baking powder, and the egg.

Divide the mixture into 6 equal portions and roll to form into balls.

Transfer to the baking sheet and bake in the preheated oven until golden brown for about 20 minutes.

Transfer to a platter to cool before serving.

STORAGE: Store in an airtight container in the fridge for up to 4 days or in the freezer for up to 1 month.

REHEAT: Microwave, covered, until it reaches the desired temperature.

SERVE IT WITH: To make this a complete meal, serve with a cup of plain yogurt and a green salad.

PER SERVING

calories: 515 | fat: 46.2g | total carbs: 5.2g | fiber: 2.0g | protein: 21.2g

VEGETABLES & SALADS

Lemony Brussels Sprout Salad with Spicy Almond

Macros: Fat: 90% | Protein: 9% | Carb: 1%

Prep time: 10 minutes | Cook time: 10 minutes | Serves 4

Quick and easy making roasted keto Brussels sprout salad flavored with lemon can be your all-time favorite side dish. To add up its delicacy, a combination of different seeds roasted under moderate temperature and spiced in chili paste make all the differences. Try to toss with dried cranberries for a different flavor. No doubt, it is a holiday salad.

FOR SPICY ALMOND AND SEED MIX:

- 1 tablespoon olive oil or refined coconut oil
- 1 teaspoon chili paste
- 2ounces (57 g) almond
- 1 ounce (28 g) pumpkin seeds
- 1 ounce (28 g) sunflower seeds
- ½ teaspoon crushed fennel seeds or ground cumin
- ¼ teaspoon salt

FOR BRUSSELS SPROUT SALAD:

- 1 pound (454 g) Brussels sprouts, trimmed and rinsed
- 2 tablespoons lemon juice and zest
- ½ cup virgin olive oil
- ¼ teaspoon pepper

- ¼ teaspoon salt

MAKE SPICY ALMOND AND SEED MIX:

In a large frying pan, pour the oil of your preference and bring low- medium heat. When the oil becomes hot, add chili and sauté for 1 minute, mix in the almond and all the seeds, and continue stirring.

Add salt and sauté for 10 minutes or until the fragrant starts to emanate.

Make sure not to burn the almonds and seeds.

Set aside until ready to serve.

MAKE BRUSSELS SPROUT SALAD:

Finely grate the Brussels sprouts with a food processor and reserve in a medium salad bowl.

In a small bowl, combine lemon juice, lemon zest, olive oil, pepper, and salt. Pour them over the grated Brussels sprouts and gently mix.

Wrap the bowl in plastic and refrigerate marinate for 10 minutes.

Serve the Brussels sprouts salad with spicy almond and seed mix on top.

STORAGE: The salad can refrigerate in a tight container for an extended shelve life. You can use it for 4 to 5 days if refrigerated properly. Take out only the required quantity at least 10 minutes before you are ready to serve.

SERVE IT WITH: It is an ideal side dish along with roasted / baked fish, meat, or chicken.

PER SERVING

calories: 457 | fat: 45.2g | total carbs: 9.1g | fiber: 7.9g | protein: 10.8g

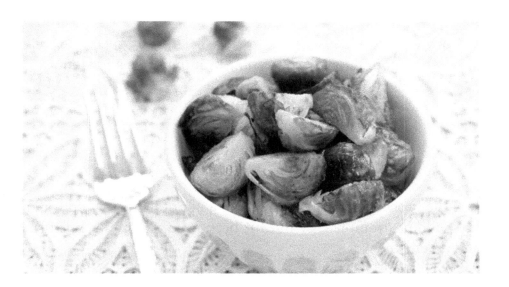

Easy Broccoli and Dill Salad

Macros: Fat: 94% | Protein: 4% | Carb: 2%

Prep time: 5 minutes | Cook time: 5 minutes | Serves 4

Think about a yummy salad that can make within moments. The salad made out of garden-fresh broccoli and dill shall remain in your heart as a staple side dish. You can easily make some variation, that can satisfy your imagination. Try using cauliflower and Brussels sprouts instead of broccoli or use a mix of all these ingredients proportionately.

- 1 pound (454 g) broccoli, cut into florets and stems
- ¾ cup fresh dill
- 1 cup keto-friendly mayonnaise
- ½ teaspoon ground pepper
- ½ teaspoon salt

Boil the broccoli florets and stems in a pot of lightly salted water for about 5 minutes, or until it becomes fork-tender but firm and greenish.

Using a colander, drain the broccoli then put it in a medium bowl. Add the fresh dill, mayonnaise and mix gently. Lightly season with pepper and salt before serving.

STORAGE: For a long day of usage, refrigerate the salad in a tight container. You can use it for 4 to 5 days if you freeze it properly. Scoop out only the required portion 10 minutes before serving.

SERVE IT WITH: It is delicious if served along with baked chicken, meat, or fish.

PER SERVING

calories: 406 | fat: 42.4g | total carbs: 4.9g | fiber: 3.1g | protein: 4.3g

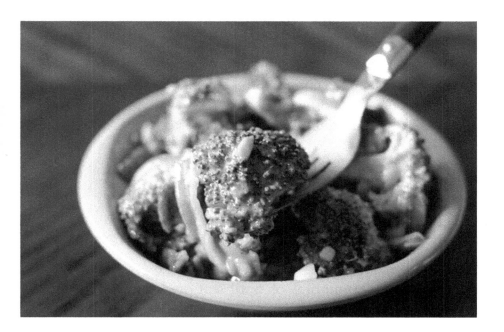

Mushroom Pizzas with Tomato Slices

Macros: Fat 71% | Protein 19% | Carbs 10%

Prep time: 15 minutes | Cook time: 5 minutes | Serves 4

Every mushroom's small pizza is a neat method to bring the inspirations together when making a thoughtful dish. You can try to change the ingredients of making such kind of pizzas, the holders can be different, and the stuffs can be different.

- 4 large portobello mushrooms, stems removed
- ¼ cup olive oil
- 1 medium tometo, cut into 4 slices
- 2 teaspoons chopped fresh basil
- 1 teaspoon minced garlic
- 1 cup shredded Mozzarella cheese

Preheat the oven to 450°F (235°C).

Arrange the mushrooms in an aluminum foil-lined baking sheet, gill side down, then brush with olive oil on all sides gently.

Place the baking sheet in the preheated oven, broil the mushrooms for 2 minutes or until soft, and then flip and broil for another 1 minute.

Make the mushroom pizza: Top each mushroom with a tomato slice, basil, minced garlic, and shredded cheese. Place the sheet back to the oven and broil for 1 minute more or until the cheese melts.

Remove the mushroom pizzas from the oven and serve warm.

STORAGE: Store in an airtight container in the fridge for up to 10 days or in

 the freezer for up to 1 month.

REHEAT: Microwave, covered, until the desired temperature is reached or reheat in a frying pan or air fryer / instant pot, covered, on medium.

SERVE IT WITH: To make this a complete meal, you can serve this dish with roasted asparagus or roasted Brussels sprouts.

PER SERVING

calories: 252 | fat: 20.1g | total carbs: 7.1g | fiber: 3.2g | protein: 14.1g

Easy Asparagus with Walnuts

Prep time: 10 minutes | Cook time: 5 minutes | Serves 4 Macros: Fat 81% | Protein 9% | Carbs 10%

The walnut itself has plenty of necessary nutrients for the human body. The

group of asparagus and walnuts is relatively a simple but different combination. So you can always find some chance to try it with your idea.

- 12 ounces (340 g) asparagus, woody ends trimmed
- ¼ cup chopped walnuts
- 1½ tablespoons olive oil
- Sea salt and freshly ground pepper, to taste

Heat the olive oil in a nonstick skillet over medium-high heat.

Add the asparagus and sauté for 5 minutes or until soft, then sprinkle with salt, and ground black pepper.

Turn the heat off. Add the walnuts and sauté to combine well.

Serve warm on a platter.

STORAGE: Store in an airtight container in the fridge for at least days or in the freezer for up to two weeks.

REHEAT: Microwave, covered, until the desired temperature is reached or reheat in a frying pan or instant pot, covered, on medium.

SERVE IT WITH: You can top the asparagus with blue cheese on the last minute of cooking time and cook until the cheese melts. It would increase the flavor of the asparagus.

PER SERVING

calories: 126 | fat: 12.2g | total carbs: 4.0g | fiber: 2.1g | protein: 1.3g

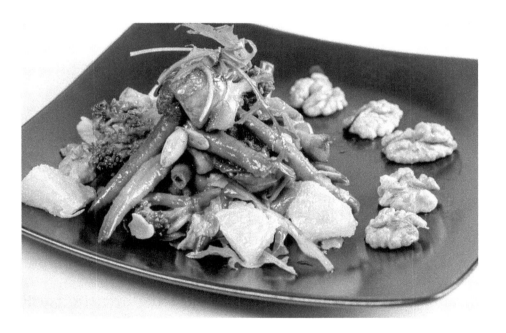

Flaxseed with Olive And Tomato Focaccia

Macros: Fat 89% | Protein 9% | Carbs 2%

Prep time: 15 minutes | Cook time: 25 minutes | Serves 18

For making this recipe, there are various ways. You can choose the traditional one to leave the olive and tomato away, or you can find something more suitable to make a focaccia. Besides, this dish is very suitable for many people to enjoy, like having a party or a big family dinner.

- 1 tablespoon baking powder
- 1 tablespoon Italian seasoning
- 2 cups roughly ground flaxseeds
- 1 teaspoon finely ground gray sea salt
- 5 large eggs
- ⅓ cup refined avocado oil
- ½ cup water
- 12 grape tomatoes, halved lengthwise
- 10 pitted olives, halved lengthwise
- 18 tablespoons keto-friendly mayonnaise

Arrange a rack in the oven, and preheat the oven to 350°F (180°C). Line the parchment paper in a baking pan.

Combine the baking powder, Italian seasoning, flaxseeds, and salt in a bowl.

Break the eggs into a blender, and add the avocado oil and water. Pulse the blender for 30 seconds or until the egg mixture is bubbly.

Make the focaccia: Pour the egg mixture in the bowl of mixture, and stir to combine well. Let sit for 3 minutes.

Spread the mixture in the baking pan with a spatula to coat the bottom of the pan evenly. Press them into the mixture until they are flush with the mixture.

Arrange the pan in the preheated oven and bake for 25 minutes or until   the pan's edges are lightly browned.

Remove the focaccia from the pan and parchment paper carefully to a cooling rack, and allow to cool for 1 hour.

Serve each focaccia with 1 tablespoon of mayo on top.

STORAGE: Store in an airtight container in the fridge for up to 3 days or in the freezer for up to 1 month.

REHEAT: Microwave, covered, until the desired temperature is reached or reheat in a frying pan or instant pot, covered, on medium.

SERVE IT WITH: To make this a complete meal, you can serve this dish with zoodles and roasted Brussels sprouts.

PER SERVING

calories: 207 | fat: 20.5g | total carbs: 5.1g | fiber: 4.0g | protein: 4.6g

Low-Carb Shichimi Collard Greens with Red Onion

Macros: Fat 81% | Protein 10% | Carbs 9%

Prep time: 15 minutes | Cook time: 15 minutes | Serves 4

The greens are always friendly to the keto diet and all creatures' health, and I believe after you know about the collards, you can find more possibilities to make the trials for more vegan foods or combinations with the meats.

- ¼ cup refined avocado oil
- ½ red onion, sliced thin
- 2 bunches collard greens (18 ounces / 510 g), stems removed, roughly chopped
- 1 teaspoon apple cider vinegar
- 1 tablespoon Shichimi seasoning
- 2 tablespoons coconut aminos
- ¼ green bell pepper, sliced thin
- Finely ground gray sea salt, to taste

Heat the avocado oil in a frying pan over medium heat, then add the sliced red onion and cook over medium-low heat for 10 minutes or until golden brown.

Add the collards, vinegar, Shichimi seasoning, and coconut aminos. Put the lid on and cook for another 5 minutes or until the collards are wilted, then top with the bell pepper and gray sea salt.

Separate the cooked collards into 4 bowls and serve warm.

STORAGE: Store in an airtight container in the fridge for no more than 3 days.

REHEAT: Microwave, covered, until the desired temperature is reached or reheat in a frying pan or instant pot, covered, on medium.

SERVE IT WITH: To make this dish complete, you can top the collards with sesame seeds and serve it with roasted chicken thighs.

PER SERVING

calories: 160 | fat: 14.4g | total carbs: 8.8g | fiber: 5.2g | protein: 3.9g

Asparagus And Pork Bake

Macros: Fat 87% | Protein 10% | Carbs 3%

Prep time: 5 minutes | Cook time: 20 minutes | Serves 4

In a casserole dish, you can always find rich and substantial flavor hidden inside. The combination of pork and asparagus is quite good and nutrients for everyone. So why not give it a try, maybe this dish will enlighten you.

- 1 pound (454 g) asparagus, tough ends removed
- ½ cup roughly ground pork rinds
- 1 cup ranch dressing
- Pinch of sea salt

Preheat the oven to 375°F (190°C).

Arrange the asparagus spears in a casserole dish. Spread the pork rinds and ranch dressing over the asparagus, then season with sea salt.

Place the casserole dish in the preheated oven and bake for 18 minutes or until lightly browned.

Transfer them onto a platter and serve warm.

STORAGE: Store in an airtight container in the fridge for no more than 3 days.

REHEAT: Microwave, covered, until the desired temperature is reached or reheat in a frying pan or instant pot, covered, on medium.

SERVE IT WITH: To make this dish complete, you can top with fresh parsley and serve it with roasted chicken thighs.

Sumptuous Egg Salad

Macros: Fat 80% | Protein 18% | Carbs 2%

Prep time: 6 minutes | Cook time: 20 minutes | Serves 4

The salad is easy to make and requires very few ingredients. It has a great taste and can serve your company as well. And this salad can be served as a salad and served as a filling for an almond-flour-made sandwich bread.

- 3 cups water
- 8 eggs
- 1 teaspoon yellow mustard
- ¼ cup green onion, chopped
- ½ cup keto-friendly mayonnaise
- ¼ teaspoon paprika
- Salt and freshly ground black pepper, to taste

In a saucepan, pour water and add eggs, then bring to a boil. Allow the eggs to sit in the hot water for 12 minutes.

Transfer the eggs to a bowl of cold water. Peel and chop the eggs into chunks.

In a separate bowl, add the chopped eggs. Stir in the mustard, green onion and mayonnaise, and toss to combine well.

Add the paprika, pepper and salt and stir well. Serve immediately.

STORAGE: Store in an airtight container in the refrigerator for up to 4 days.

SERVE IT WITH: To make this a complete meal, serve it between gluten- free almond bread or coconut crackers.

PER SERVING

calories: 449 | fat: 39.9g | total carbs: 2.9g | fiber: 0.3g | protein: 18.4g

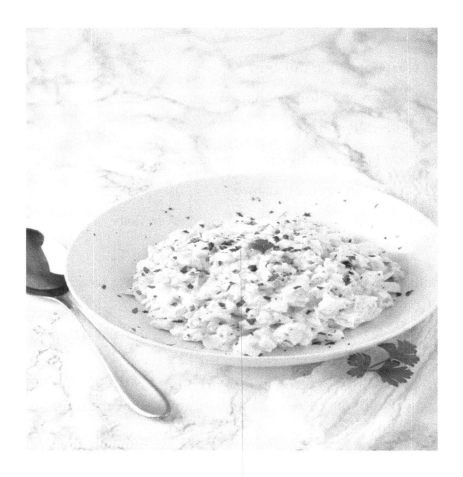

Egg Salad with Mustard Dressing

Macros: Fat 76% | Protein 20% | Carbs 4%

Prep time: 6 minutes | Cook time: 10 minutes | Serves 4

It is an interesting egg salad. The lemon's fresh vibe and the Dijon mustard tang make it a must if you love salads.

- 2½ cups water 6 eggs

DRESSING:

- 1 teaspoon Dijon mustard
- ¼ cup green onions, chopped
- ½ juiced lemon
- ¼ cup keto-friendly mayonnaise
- ½ teaspoon yellow mustard
- Salt and freshly ground black pepper, to taste

In a saucepan, pour the water and add eggs. Bring to a boil for about 10 minutes.

Transfer the eggs to a bowl of cold water. Peel and chop the eggs into ½- inch chunks. Set aside.

Make the dressing: In a medium bowl, add the Dijon mustard, green onions, lemon juice, mayonnaise, and yellow mustard and thoroughly mix.

Pour the dressing over the egg chunks and sprinkle with salt, and pepper.

Gently toss to combine well and serve.

STORAGE: Store in an airtight container in the refrigerator for up to 4 days.

SERVE IT WITH: To make this a complete meal, serve it with seared salmon fillets.

PER SERVING

calories: 293 | fat: 24.9g | total carbs: 2.8g | fiber: 0.3g | protein: 13.8g

Avocado, Cucumber and Bacon Salad

Macros: Fat 92% | Protein 1% | Carbs 6%

Prep time: 15 minutes | Cook time: 8 minutes | Serves 8

This is an extremely easy salad to prepare. It is healthy and tasty for bacon and avocado lovers. The freshness of cucumber combined with the taste of avocado will release the potential of the salad.

- 1 pound (454 g) bacon, chopped
- 1 cup cherry tomatoes, quartered
- 1 cucumber, diced
- ¼ cup rice vinegar
- Salt and freshly ground black pepper, to taste
- ½ cup fresh cilantro, chopped
- 4 green onions, chopped
- 5 avocados, peeled, pitted and diced

In a nonstick skillet over medium-high heat, add bacon and cook for 8 minutes until browned, flipping occasionally. Drain the bacon on a paper towel and crumble into small pieces. Set aside on a plate.

In a medium bowl, add tomatoes, cucumber, rice vinegar, pepper and salt.

Stir well to mix.

Fold in the bacon, cilantro, green onions, and avocado. Toss to combine well.

Divide the salad among serving plates, then serve.

STORAGE: Store in an airtight container in the refrigerator for up to 4 days.

SERVE IT WITH: To make this a complete meal, serve with buttered cod.

PER SERVING

calories: 721 | fat: 74.9g | total carbs: 12.8g | fiber: 9.1g | protein: 3.1g

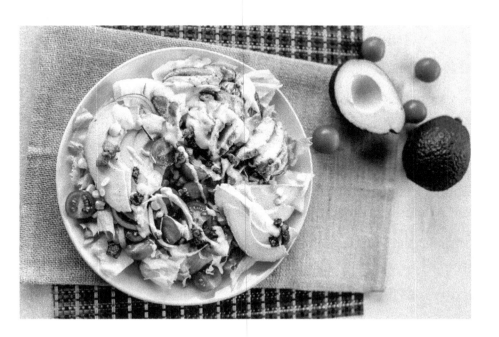

Brussels Sprouts Citrus Bacon Dressing

Macros: Fat 71% | Protein 16% | Carbs 13%

Prep time: 10 minutes | Cook time: 10 minutes | Serves 4

The Brussels sprouts with a bacon dressing is a nutritious delicacy that is easy to make. The lemon and apple cider vinegar gives it a unique flavor fusion.

- 1¼ pounds (567 g) Brussels sprouts, cut into strips
- 1 tablespoon olive oil
- 4 ounces (113 g) sliced bacon
- 3 tablespoons erythritol
- ⅓ cup apple cider vinegar
- 1 lemon, juiced
- Salt and freshly ground black pepper, to taste Cayenne pepper, to taste

In a nonstick skillet over medium heat, heat the olive oil. Add bacon and cook for 8 minutes until it buckles and curls, flipping occasionally.

Add the erythritol, apple cider vinegar, lemon juice, black pepper, salt and cayenne pepper. Stir well to mix. Reduce the heat to medium- high and cook for 1 minute more.

Transfer the bacon mixture to a large bowl and add the Brussels sprouts.

Gently toss until well combined.

Let it rest for 5 minutes and serve.

STORAGE: Store in an airtight container in the refrigerator for up to 4 days.

SERVE IT WITH: To make this a complete meal, serve with beef steak and berry smoothie.

PER SERVING

calories: 248 | fat: 15.0g | total carbs: 13.9g | fiber: 5.4g | protein: 8.4g

EXTRA KETO TREATS

Buttery Walnut Toffee Bark

Yields Provided: 24 Servings

Macro Counts for Each Serving:

- Total Net Carbs: 2 g
- Protein: 1 g
- Fat Content: 11 g
- Calories: 105

List of Ingredients:

- Butter (5 tbsp.)
- Chopped walnuts (1 cup)
- Heavy cream (5 tbsp.)
- Trim Healthy Mama Gentle Sweet or your choice sweetener (.5 cup)
- Salt (1 pinch)
- Dark chocolate - sugar-free (7 oz.)

Preparation Technique:

1. Prepare a baking pan with a layer of aluminum foil. Spritz with cooking a portion of oil spray.

2. Melt the butter using the med-low heat setting until it starts browning. Fold in the nuts and simmer until they are lightly toasted (5 min.).

3.   Add four tablespoons of cream, and sweetener. Simmer until thickened (10 min.). If needed, you can increase the heat to medium or med-high while stirring constantly.

4.   Remove and add the salt and reserved cream. Stir until smooth. Pour onto the foil-lined baking tray and refrigerate until firm to the touch (30 min.).

5.   Melt the chocolate in the microwave - stirring every thirty seconds. Pour half of the chocolate on top of the toffee.

6.   Pop into the freezer until the chocolate is solid. Flip the toffee bark and peel off the foil. Put the foil back on the tray and place the toffee on top (chocolate side down). Pour the rest of the chocolate on top. Refrigerate or freeze until firm.

7.   The filling stays soft like a caramel for the first few hours but will harden like a toffee overnight.

Chocolate Covered Cheesecake Bites

Yields Provided: 16 Servings

Macro Counts for Each Serving:

- Fat Content: 7 g

- Total Net Carbs: 2 g

- Protein: 1 g

List of Ingredients:

- Cream cheese (8 oz. - softened)

- Gentle Sweet or your choice low-carb powdered sugar (4 tbsp.)

- Heavy cream (2 tbsp.)

- Diced strawberries (1 cup fresh)

List of Ingredients - Chocolate Drizzle:

- Lily's chocolate chips (3 tbsp.)

- Melted coconut oil (1 tsp.)

Preparation Technique:

1. In a medium mixing container, whip the softened cream cheese with the sweetener and heavy cream.

2. When mixture is slightly thickened, add diced strawberries, and stir gently to mix the strawberries into the cheesecake mixture.

3. Scoop into mounds on a parchment-lined cookie sheet and place in the freezer.

4. When cheesecake bites have completely frozen, drizzle lightly using the melted chocolate mixture.

5.   To make the melted chocolate, simply microwave the chocolate chips with coconut oil in 20 to 30-second intervals, stirring well after each, until the chocolate is melted and smooth.

6.   Return chocolate drizzled cheesecake bites to the freezer to harden the chocolate.

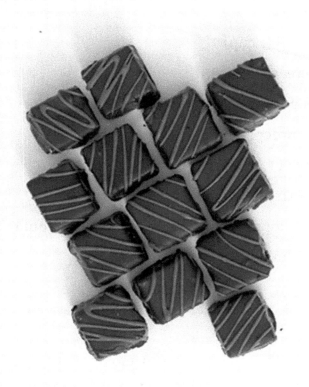

Chocolate Peanut Butter Cups

Yields Provided: 12 Servings Macro Counts for Each Serving:

- Fat Content: 26 g

- Total Net Carbs: 2.2 g

- Protein: 3.4g

- Calories: 246

List of Ingredients:

- Coconut oil (1 cup)

- Heavy cream (2 tbsp.)

- Natural peanut butter or another butter (.5 cup)

- Cocoa powder (1 tbsp.)

- Kosher salt (.25 tsp.)

- Vanilla extract (.25 tsp.)

- Roasted chopped salted peanuts or another nut (1 oz.)

Preparation Technique:

1.   Use the low setting on the stovetop to prepare a saucepan with the coconut oil. Once it's hot (3-5 min.), stir in the rest of the fixings.

2.   Pour into the silicone muffin molds or use an ice tray. Sprinkle with the nuts and put them on a baking tray.

3.   Freeze until the mixture is firm or for about one hour. Pop-out the peanut butter cups out of the molds and place them in an airtight container to enjoy.

Cream Cheese Truffles

Yields Provided: 24 Servings

Macro Counts for Each Serving:

- Fat Content: 7 g

- Total Net Carbs: 1.67 g

- Protein: 1.23 g

- Calories: 72.7

List of Ingredients:

- Softened cream cheese (16 oz.)

- Unsweetened cocoa powder - divided (.5 cup)

- Swerve confectioners (4 tbsp.)

- Liquid Stevia (.25 tsp.

- Rum extract (.5 tsp.)

- Instant coffee (1 tbsp.)

- Water (2 tbsp.)

- Heavy whipping cream (1 tbsp.)

- Paper candy cups - for serving (24)

Preparation Technique:

1.   Combine all of the fixings (set aside .25 cup of cocoa powder).

2.   Blend well with a hand mixer. Chill in the fridge for about 30 minutes.

3.   Dust the countertop with the rest of the cocoa powder.

4.   Roll out heaping tablespoons of the mixture in your hands to form about 24 balls. Roll the balls through the powder and place into individual candy cups.

5.   Chill for another hour before serving.

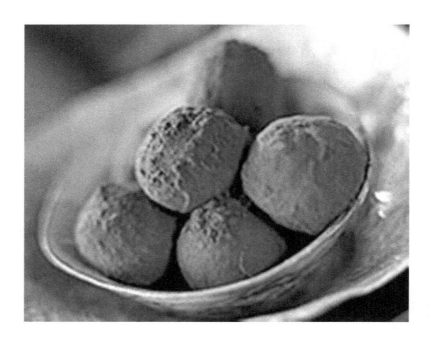

CPSIA information can be obtained
at www.ICGtesting.com
Printed in the USA
BVHW061520250321
603414BV00002B/539